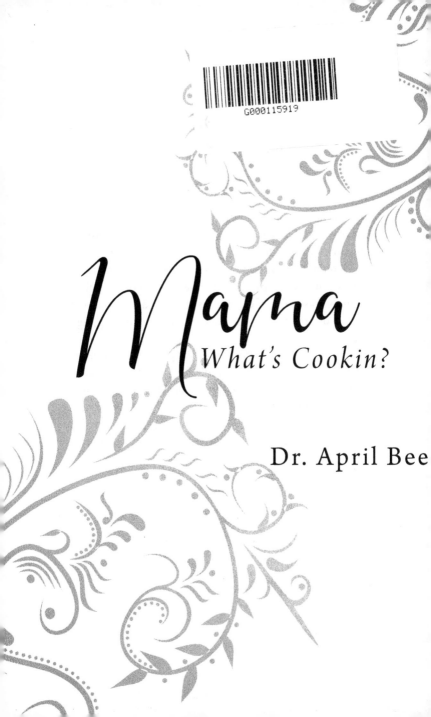

Mama
What's Cookin?

Dr. April Bee

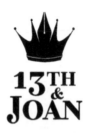

13TH & JOAN

For permission requests, write to the publisher, addressed "Attention: Permissions Coordinator," 205 N. Michigan Avenue, Suite #810, Chicago, IL 60601. 13th & Joan books may be purchased for educational, business or sales promotional use. For information, please email the Sales Department at sales@13thandjoan.com.

Printed in the U. S. A.

First Printing, July 2022.

Library of Congress Cataloging-in-Publication Data has been applied for.

ISBN: 978-1-953156-10-5

These stories are not only dedicated to my mama, but dedicated to the freedom of the truths of her story. This is dedicated to the fullness of her life and motherhood, and anything that anyone once tried to silence or avoid. This is dedicated to our lineage and legacy, our healing, our growth, our joy. This is dedicated to God's aligned purpose for everything that has led to this moment in ensuring that your truths ring into the atmosphere. This is dedicated to every smile that may have held back tears, and every brave moment that may have held back fears. This is for the true continuance of your beauty, Cindy Rae.

"Despite everything, no one can dictate
who you are to other people."

—Prince

Contents

Preface 1

Introduction 7

Mama's Wash Day 13

Say Your Prayers, Mama 23

"She's Not a Real Mom" 33

Eww, Mama Drools... 43

Mama's Sunshine.. 53

Mama, Let's Cry Together....................................... 63

Mama's Strawberry Cake 73

The RV Trip with Mama 83

Mama Loves the Bad Boys 93

Preface

1 AM MY MAMA'S DAUGHTER.

I am strong, sensitive, sweet, and sultry. I am light in the space of my darkest times. I am a story that is waiting to be told. I am a collection of smiles, laughs, and positive moments. I am a recollection of pain, endurance and perseverance. I am oppositional in fear and driven in love. I am wrapped genuinely and authentically, ready to unravel into a vulnerable endeavor of freedom and self-acceptance. I am beauty waiting to be revealed. I truly am my mama, Cindy Rae.

Cindy Rae, also known as mama, was a beautiful, big-hearted, and bright woman from the southern parts of Memphis. She was full of warmth and love that resonated with every soul that she encountered. She was the oldest of three girls, which put her in a place of being a caretaker for them. Her mom, who is my grandma, was a young Ph.D student building her career with her husband, my grandpa. They lived in Worthington, Ohio, a suburb of Columbus. There she radiated in her intelligence and athleticism which landed her the opportunity to graduate high school early and play for The Ohio State women's basketball team at the age of 16. At a point, she started to fall a lot during practice as well as struggled with balance. She wasn't fully sure what was causing this, but it got in the way of her opportunities to focus in school and to play basketball. After a couple of years of doctor's visits, she was given the news that she had been diagnosed with Multiple Sclerosis (MS).

Multiple Sclerosis is an interesting disease because it can manifest quite differently in each person. There are different types of MS and different ways that each type presents itself. Mama began with Primary Progressive MS (PPMS) and then progressed into Secondary Progressive MS (SPMS), which means there was an initial response in her nervous system and then the symptoms progressed into a disability which then stables out as non-active relapses with or without progression. Basically, mama went from falling time to time, to walking with a cane, to walking with a walker, to needing a wheelchair, to becoming fully bedridden. She went from fully being able to speak, to little speech that is slurred, to not being able to speak at all. Mama birthed me in the middle of this progression at the stage of being in a wheelchair and having limited motor skills. I proudly came out four days late at ten heavy pounds–natural birth. Mama could hold and hug me as a baby and occasionally crawl around with me. I have faint memories of her being able to fully call my name as an explorative two-year old and a few words here and there shortly after. But, as I continued to get older, she lost her motor skills to interact with me in the same manner.

Therefore, I had the unique experience of growing up with a mama who was fully bed-written and disabled. We had the opportunity to manually wash her daily. We had the opportunity to cut up the back of her shirts and slide them on her body daily. We had the opportunity to feed her and give her water through a stomach tube. The opportunity to wipe off her sweat if she got hot and warm her up if she got cold. The opportunity to care for her at any given time and make sure that she was always as healthy as possible. This was our reality. Over the years, there were plenty of reminders that the world saw her differently than I saw her. People continued to see her disability, which of course was evident and present. Yet, it somehow seemed like a struggle for people to see her as a functional human being.

To be transparent, I internalized those thoughts as well. I didn't know how to fully take in the fact that my mother could not move, could not fully talk, run around, hold me, cook, drive, or anything else that the other parents did. I had to force myself to remember to tell mama good-bye before school and goodnight at night. I had to remember to still talk to her, even if she couldn't talk back. With this, I also saw how much of a mama she truly was. I saw that she made me happier than any other person in this world. I saw that she created warmth, peace, and safety with just her presence. She demonstrated womanhood and instilled the greatest values of life within. She was such a competent and functioning mama.

I honestly am still learning to unpack on how to navigate if I was truly traumatized by my mom, or if I was just seeing trauma through the projection of others. I often internalized the limited perceptions of others without recognizing that most people have a limited capacity on understanding how someone can be able and disable simultaneously. I never conceptualized how vulnerable it may feel for someone to see the full human in someone who lacks critical physical abilities. To look at a person restricted in motion and imagine that they are filled with boundless emotion. To know that the way you look at them could trigger them to either laugh or cry, but not have the ability to show it. The perceptions in media have heavily influenced how people interpret situations with mama. To know that cinematic depictions of disability cast it only as an inability to live a fullness of life assured others that mama was merely a collection of cells existing in a space with a disabled body and mind.

Therefore, I am overly excited to finally share the truth of mama's ability to be a mama. Although it had its obvious limitations, there were way more liberations. I learned more from her than I learned from any woman in my life, so it feels truly special to share the fullness of motherhood beyond physical expectations. This has been such a vulnerable journey of unpacking and healing. Prepare for a journey of a plethora of genuine emotions and experiences that awaken and expand the most ordinary thoughts of an extraordinary woman— Cindy Rae.

Introduction

S0, YOU'RE PROBABLY WONDERING WHY THIS IS called, Mama, What's Cookin'?

Well, although there were many experiences of such, there is one specific experience that I remember from childhood that best highlights the complexity and charm of mama being mama. This story falls into the common occurrences of interacting with mama, and the moment I realized that there were two different realities of her existence.

One day, Daddy and I were cooking in the kitchen and making soul food. At this time, we lived with my maternal grandma and grandpa to help with taking care of mama. We had lived with them for the majority of my childhood until I moved away to college. It always brought an interesting twist to the household dynamics living with my grandparents and parents. Sometimes, my grandparents would come down and visit with mama for a little bit. They would watch TV or talk to her about life, or just sit with her and enjoy her presence. Since she was not able to say much, just experiencing her presence was always an abundance of peace. My mama's progression of MS was so far that she had very slurred and delayed speech. Therefore, it was sometimes difficult to understand what she was saying, and she didn't often speak. Nonetheless, I always somehow knew her exact words. So, my grandma was sitting with her and talking to her about a few different things. Mama then replied back in the rarest of moments. She said an entire sentence.

I then heard my grandma scream, "April! Please come here!" and so I scurried into the room in urgency. I met her with a look of frustration as she was continuously asking mama to repeat herself, as mama kept kindly repeating an exact sentence. Grandma then abruptly stopped the attempts and requested,

"Tell me what she is trying to say." So, I turned to mama in slight confusion and said, "Mama, what's up?" She slurred, "something smells really good—what's cookin'?" I got excited and a smile broadened across my face because it is not often at all that mama ever talks, and I rarely hear her say an entire sentence. I then played with her and said, "What's cookin', mama!?" She smiled back and guessed, "chicken?" I then cheered for her, and explained, "Yes! Daddy and I are cooking collard greens, shake and bake chicken, and cornbread!" She smiled wide and slurred, "I can't wait!" I could tell that my grandma was slightly bothered that she could not understand her daughter's words. She asked, "wow—how did you know what she said so quickly?" I said, "it really sounded clear to me."

I then realized in that moment our reality. It was difficult for others to understand mama. No matter how crystal clear it can be shown to me, it may be completely blurry to others. Mama couldn't be heard—literally and metaphorically. Even the closest people, family included, may not have the capacity to experience mama in her fullness. For some, it may hurt too much or trigger them. For some, it may be too much energy. For some, they just may not know how. Some will struggle to share the bond that we have. They may not even fully understand it, receive it, or accept it. Some will struggle to understand what it is like to be stuck in a bed all of the time, and people do not understand your simplest expressions—sometimes, not even your mother. And, no one will understand how hard it is to see your mom as just a weak disabled person, when I always have seen a superwoman.

It was hard for me to understand what everyone else couldn't see. Perhaps I normalized this life experience so much that I haven't recognized how abnormal it really is. I saw myself having a fully capable mama with a few things missing, but isn't that every human? I am not a great singer, I'm not the tallest, I'm only right-handed, I was clumsy, I couldn't climb a tree, I didn't run the fastest although very athletic. See? I'm missing some physical attributes too, just like mama. Why does hers make her less human to the world? Sometimes I can't tell people when I'm in pain, or when I am afraid. I can't always express when something bothers me or even when I am in the greatest of excitement. Sometimes I am sad and I just don't know why. See? I sometimes cannot express myself, just like mama. Why does hers make her less human to the world? Why can't everyone hear her words? Why can't everyone understand her cries? Isn't mama a mama too?

This cooking experience robbed my innocence of the truth on who mama was and what she could do. I would spend the continuing years unpacking and navigating how mama was now perceived to the world. I was protected in this bubble of life where mama was perfect and perfectly fine, while just doing physically unique things. But now, I had to come to terms on the disability that others saw and experienced, while clenching tight to the full ability of her that I treasured.

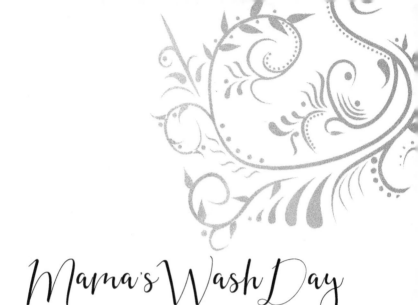

Mama's Wash Day

ONE OF THE MOST JOYFUL MOMENTS THAT I got to share with mama was washing her beautiful hair. Since she was bedridden, we had to wash her hair in a non-traditional way. Even though it was uncommon, I always looked forward to the adventure of nurturing and cleansing her beautiful locks. When it was that time of the week, I would beg my daddy to let me wash her beautiful hair. I know that he was always hesitant because I was a small child asking to play in water but to me this wasn't a moment of play—this was an intimate experience to endeavor into the limited ways that I could take care of mama. I couldn't wait to run my fingers through her hair and massage through the mirror image of my own mahogany crown. I would attempt to wash it every day, if I could.

I think this excitement stems from the exceptional opportunity to tangibly experience the beauty of mama despite her condition. It was the opportunity that while seeing a body immobile in a motorized bed with back-cut shirts and tubes injected in multiple uncomfortable areas, her crown remained so luxurious and full. It was the piece of her that I hoped that people could at least give proper acknowledgement to while being so uncomfortable with the rest of her body. Although I saw her entire body as an absolutely beautiful masterpiece, I recognized that her unique structure may be difficult to conceptualize.

I also loved mama's hair because it was the one thing that we could share about our bodies—we had the same, functioning hair. We both had the same hair pattern, and often wore it in similar styles. It felt the same. It looked the same— she just had a lot of maturity and healthiness in her tresses compared to my kid-like fuzzes. It was my connection—my moment to contribute to loving on mama, and in some ways, directly loving on myself. Sometimes, one of the only times that I could truly experience intimacy with mama was through washing her hair since we weren't able to physically share too much more. Nonetheless, it was a reminder that in the midst of her difficulties, there was still a moment of beauty and joy—simply in the crown of mama's hair. Truly, this day left me elated each time.

Mama's hair was soft and freeing with wide and open curls that bounced into the palms of my hands like the boundless and rolling ocean waves. Her hair was a soft ebony but shined as a hue of dark brown in the brightest sunlight to match her chocolate eyes. Her hair never seemed tangled as each spiral stood in its own elegance above the frame of her head. The sweet aroma of oils bring a tender sleek texture to her curls as they wrap around my fingers like a coiled blanket. I loved rubbing the pull of her ponytail to feel the patterns of her rippling curls pulled all into one fruitful crown upon the top of head. You could only imagine the eloquent serenity of tussling her coils.

I wake up earlier than normal for mama's wash day, as I am anxiously awaiting the serendipitous joy that mama and I will share. I grab the blow-up water reserve used to wash mama's hair from the top shelf in the bathroom. Balancing on my tippy toes upon the footstool, I rest the water reserve upon my head like a droopy wig. I loved smelling the lingering aroma of shampoo in the reserve as I stepped down and walked into our bedroom. I then put the reserve down to blow it up until it becomes an inflated pillow and plug it tightly. After daddy finishes cleaning mama up for the day, he says "it's time", with a reserved expression of excitement. I scurry over and then take the water reserve from the top of my head to the underneath of mama's. We slowly let her bed down so that it flattened, just as a beauty salon. My daddy then runs to the bathroom to get the large pink bowl and fill it up with warm water. He also grabs the Sulfur 8 Shampoo, conditioner, a large pink comb that is strong but highly worn down, and a large towel to ensure mama doesn't need yet another bath. In the meantime, I gently took the ponytail holder and unlocked it from her coils to free her hair. Her curls opened up and bounced around the water reserve, and we both softly smiled. I would then gently separate her hair and run my fingers through to catch the smallest snags. Her hair was like a soft pillow—gave me comfort and safety no matter what I was going through.

Daddy quickly came back juggling all of the things needed to wash mama's hair. He pours the semi-steaming water into the reserve, fogging up his glasses. I watch her curls flatten into synchronized ripples like the shore of a beach during a high tide. I anxiously stick my fingers into her dampened hair while bravely bearing the unpleasant sensation of the heated water. I softly used the knubs of my fingers to massage her scalp in circular rotations and then switched to pressing in with my nails for a tingling sensation. Daddy then squeezed a sizable amount of Sulfur 8 Shampoo atop a few curls and we began to massage it in her hair together. We laughed when a couple of bubbles would fly upon our faces, or even on mama's face. Sometimes she would laugh too. I would occasionally look up at daddy and I was always inspired by the presence of love and joy in his eyes as he washes his beautiful wife's hair. Daddy always made taking care of my mama seem like the greatest and easiest thing in the world to do. He loved her so much, and I could especially tell in the moment his sheer joy of connection between the three of us, all over mama's hair. I allowed the shampoo to toil in my nail buds as I looked down and continued to scrub. I loved how the scent of Sulfur 8 shampoo filled every follicle of my nose—a scent that will forever reside in me. We then rinsed the water around in the reserve and lifted her head gently to wash out all of the shampoo. Daddy would then squeeze a dollop of conditioner into his hands and rub it through her cleansed coils. The thin yellow conditioner had a unique smell that seemed to make my eyes water, so I would focus on playing with mama's hair to distract the smell. I would then grab the pink comb, and gently comb out different sections of her curls. As I have also experienced this pink comb, I think about the toiling pains it has caused while getting my hair done. Contrary to my experiences, mama doesn't even budge when I comb her hair. As a young girl, I knew that I wasn't as gentle at times and pulled a little too hard to detangle, but she would lie there and continue to smile as if this experience is the greatest on this earth. I know for me, it was. Oh, how something so simple could be so joyous.

After the very last rinse, it was time to drain the water from her reserve. This was the much-dreaded sign that wash day was almost over. The reserve came with a tube on the side that pushes out to allow the water to safely drain into a container. We would pour the water into the original pink bowl as we gently and firmly squeeze any excess water from mama's hair. I then had the greatest task of combing through, oiling, and braiding mama's hair. I would take each wet piece of hair and rub the grease through it, stretching each piece back as far as it goes just to let go and watch the curls bounce back into place. Her coils are now filled with even more shine and luster than before. I continued to press through oiling her hair as the burn of the grease intoxicated my eyes. I comb her hair for the final time and begin to separate parts to braid. From age four and beyond, I enjoyed braiding mama's hair so much because it was so beautiful, and I loved taking part in helping her to feel beautiful.

As I got older, mama's wash days were always still meaningful but didn't always have the same flare. Sometimes I would wash her hair alone if daddy had work or school. There would be times where I wouldn't get to wash her hair much because her nursing aid would wash her hair for us. It was such an enjoyable experience for anyone who touched her precious locks. It would often excite me when I came home from school and saw mama with a beautiful new hair-do and see the smile on her face.

As mama's MS symptoms progressed, it also impacted the health of her hair. Although her body was transitioning so much, her beautiful coils remained strong, bountiful, and full of luster. It was another reminder that through the most difficult things, her beauty would always persevere through. Her consistency in such beauty gave me hope that through the toughest moments of life, there will always be something bright and beautiful, just like mama. As I matured, I was so warmed to know that my hair would grow into looking like hers. We had similar locks, curls, and coils and I would always find ways to style it like hers until I started getting perms. I was so glad that I still had mama's hair to play with since my hair had a new texture. She would still smile when I touched her now fuzzed but rippled edges, and would massage my long nails throughout her sensitive scalp. I would occasionally still braid her hair if her nurses hadn't touched it up and made sure to gently arrange her large puff as if they were a beautiful bouquet of flowers in a vase.

Whenever we visited mama in the nursing home, daddy would still always stroke her hair while looking into her eyes and telling her how much he loved her, and she always looked so connected. I would also sometimes come in and just play with her hair as I sat and talked to her. My favorite thing was to twirl her long edges around my pinky finger and then release to watch a coil spring back. Sometimes I would just play with her hair as we prayed or as we watched TV. It became a comforting coping mechanism not only with mama, but with other people I felt close to. I will never forget the touch of mama's hair and the energy I experienced from her crown to my roots. I sometimes randomly massage my own hair hoping to feel the soft and enriching feeling mama's hair gave to me. It truly brought happiness to know that the blessing of mama's coils would always keep us connected as a family through any season of life.

Currently, my wash days look quite similar to mama's. I am excited to wake up, and gather all the supplies needed to make this task successful. I now turn on some of mama's favorite songs, or just a podcast if I'm in a different mood. I let my wild curls down to fall everywhere in their unique and bold form and go through the entire wash process. I play in my similarly formed curls, rubbing my fingerprints along the soft, smooth texture. Rustling around in the lather, I reach deeply into my scalp and massage in circles to gently feel the scratching sensation of our similar scalps. I inhale the distinct scent of my shampoo and find gratitude in the sensory experience of mama's presence. I pull upon each coil with my wrinkled fingers, combing them one by one, and sometimes playing with them. I gently smile when I feel the familiar sensations of mama's hair within my tresses, as if I'm now washing her crown. Although it is not the same pink comb, I do have a pink comb to detangle my hair. Pulling each section of hair until all of the curls spring back into the unified positions. I rinse, dry, and slowly style. It feels so comforting to know that wash day will always continue on and that I can have this heartwarming experience to pass along over the years and generations.

I'm off to prepare for my next wash day.

Say Your Prayers, Mama

*"Dear Lord, we thank you for another day, and the
blessings you bestowed upon us. Please watch over
our family, friends, and people all around the world.
Please help us to grow happy, healthy, and strong."*

THESE WERE THE OPENING WORDS OF THE
repeated nightly prayer that we had with mama
each night. I was blessed to come from a family
unit where we would take intentional time to
pray together. This practice carried through

into my adulthood. and truly impacted my outlook on connectedness and spirituality. Daddy took this seriously and made sure that no matter the circumstance, we would find time to pray, daily. With the things he had overcome, the current things mama was overcoming, and with me growing as a child, we saw the importance of consistent prayer. I also learned the depth and power of connecting spiritually as a family, and what it meant to create a bond with mama in the Spirit—something that lasts further than the years we would be on this Earth. We would start each morning by saying a very short prayer to start the day. After the 64-inch TV was on all night, daddy would grab the large gray remote with opaque blue buttons and press the "OFF" button, which was the sign that we were about to pray together. Daddy would grab my hand and then mama's hand, and then I would grab mama's other soft, dainty hand.

Mama had slurred and delayed speech, as well as difficulty with memory recall as a symptom of the severity of her MS, so sometimes it would be hard for her to recall what exact words we said every night during the prayer. MS directly affects how the messages travel from your brain and down your spinal. When there is lots of scarring on the myelin (the things that protect the message) then sometimes those messages don't reach their destination on time or at all. Therefore, daddy and I would sometimes have to feed her words during our daily and nightly prayers. This added an extra special tone to the experience of praying with my family because it taught us patience and humility in the midst of humbling ourselves before God. Sometimes, I believe God gave us this unique assignment to continuously strengthen us as a family even with our large hosts of brokenness. It was fun to help mama say the words as I was learning the words myself.

Sometimes daddy would sit and allow her to figure the words out on her own so he could keep her cognitive function strengthened. I would sit there with my eyes closed and hands squeezed tightly, patiently (or impatiently) waiting for mama to recall the words. I would sometimes peek an eye open to see if there was any way to expedite this process due to my growing hunger. Nonetheless, I wanted mama to recall the words and feel like she had enough time to do so. But, sometimes she just couldn't. So, for most of the prayers we would close our eyes. Daddy begins by first saying the words, and waiting for mama to repeat along–feeding them to her so that she can say them with him, and I can quietly follow along. We would say collectively:

"Dear Lord, we thank you for waking us up today, into another beautiful morning. I ask that you please watch over our family and friends coast, and people all around the world. Please help us to grow happy, healthy, and strong. All these things, I pray, in the name of Jesus Christ, Lord and Savior, Amen."

At times, whether in the morning or in the evening, I would be too sleepy to fully participate. So, I would sometimes cut out on a few words of the prayer. If I did, daddy would firmly squeeze my hand to ensure that I was awake and I would quickly jump back in before the entire prayer was finished. As a kid, it seemed redundant and annoying to pray every single morning and evening over and over. I didn't fully understand the point. Sometimes, I would hide the TV remote so daddy can't cut it off and therefore we didn't have to pray. Of course, there were power buttons on the TV so it would cut off eventually and we would be back in routine once again. I didn't necessarily dislike prayer, I just didn't like how long it took and that it always had to come right before eating food! Because of my dismay towards these arrangements, I did inquire to daddy as to why we pray daily, especially since it's the exact same prayer. "Didn't God hear us the first time?" Daddy firmly and wisely reminded me of the circumstances we were in—mama was completely disabled and daddy was recovering from a lot of hardships in his past. He knows it is only a blessing from God that we are even here together as a family with a roof over our head, and healthy enough to spend everyday together. He knows that only God could sustain us from how difficult things were for us and to keep us on the right path towards a brighter future. We couldn't just call on God once, but had to walk with Him daily to truly receive the protection that we needed as a family. He knew that the only person that can help protect us through this life is God. As an adult, I see how well those prayers truly worked.

Our nightly prayers were a little longer, so we would recite it a little differently. After cooking an amazing meal, daddy would ask me to lay out a rectangular brown towel with black and cream patterns. We would put this on the bed so we could all eat together as a family beside mama in the bedroom. As a child, my daddy would slide his bed closer to her bed so that we would all be in close proximity. Daddy would then bring the food in the room and place it on the towel. After having everything set, we would turn off the TV, close our eyes and prepare for prayer. Mama and I would say the first few lines of the prayer, which sounds a lot like our morning prayer:

"Dear Lord, we thank you for another day, and the blessings you bestowed upon us. Please watch over our family, friends, and people all around the world. Please help us to grow happy, healthy, and strong."

From there, my daddy would go into his part of the prayer. He would pray for each family member, and for our personal health. He would pray for us to remain safe and for me to grow up well. He would pray for our sins that we have committed and the ones to come. He would especially pray for mama's health. This prayer lasted about five minutes long each night, so as a kid I would again check out time to time, allow the highly intoxicating aroma of the food to take me away, think about what cool thing happened at school today, or what game I'm going to play after dinner and before bed. He would occasionally rub my hands if I would become fidgety to remind me to focus back into the prayer. I sometimes allowed my mind to wander in thinking about how many of our prayers came true that we have spoken. I thought of how healthy everyone around us has been, how I was growing up nicely, and how even in the hardest moments of life, everyone seemed to be doing well. I then took this moment to daydream and think about my life in the future where mama would be fully healthy again. She would be able to walk, and fully talk. She would be able to go outside and play basketball with me and come to all of my games. She would help me get dressed for my wedding and put on my earrings before I go down the aisle. She would come visit me or we would go on trips together with my girls and just laugh and enjoy life. She wouldn't be sick anymore. I then became grateful for taking so much time to pray, and saw a charge to take it more seriously. I prayed harder because I wanted to make sure that everything came true with mama. I even started to find the value in praying on my own.

One thing that I did honor about our prayers is that no matter where we were—the hospital, the nursing home, or a family member's house—we were going to pray together. Even if I was staying the night at someone's house, daddy would make sure that we prayed as a family before I left. Even if we were in a rush, or if we got to the nursing home too late to visit mama, we would still make time for prayer. It felt slightly embarrassing most times, especially in public areas where people walked in, but in hindsight, it set a precedent to the world and to God that we were dedicated to protecting our family with the power of prayer, every single day. We said the exact same words every single time, but it always sat so deeply in my heart.

As we began to wrap up the prayer we finished with saying the same closing lines together:

> *"All these things,*
> *I pray,*
> *In the name of Jesus Christ,*
> *Lord Savior,*
> *Amen."*

Daddy and I always rejoiced at the times when mama was able to say the entire ending of the prayer with us. He would exclaim with so much gratitude in his heart and voice:

"Yay, mama--you said it!"

She always smiled softly to us.

Over the years, mama's ability to fully finish the prayer diminished because of her increasing MS symptoms. There were times when daddy would feed her words, and she just was not able to say it back anymore. I remember sometimes peeking open an eye to look at daddy's face in response to her not being able to repeat his words back. I saw a disturbing numbed expression of worry with a glaze of pain. To the common eye and interpretation it looked like anger, but I knew daddy. He wasn't angry at mama. He didn't know how to process her shift in health each day. I didn't either. It was a difficult dissonance to accept—praying to God for good health over family and friends (including mama) while mama was decreasing in health right before our eyes. Nonetheless, I am affirmed that those daily prayers allowed her to live years beyond the doctor's expectations and keeps my daddy and I healthy throughout this day.

I had to learn over time how valuable it was to include mama in our prayers, even if and when she couldn't talk. I also had to allow myself to learn how necessary it was to pray for her—literally. I was her voice when she could no longer speak. I was her only child. I was the carrier of her spiritual needs and the intercessor for her health. Although that was a large responsibility as just a child, I acknowledge that it was my greatest gift for her and the most special form of worship— being the praying voice for mama. I recognized that although we repeated these words each night, it was also a meditation upon our heart and spirit. We had to repeat it multiple times to truly believe in the fight we have taken on, and that we would be victorious. We had to believe that together, as a family, we would conquer the hardest times and be consistent in it. Even in our fear and worry, we would always grab mama's soft and dainty hands, and pray together. With that, I am grateful that God used me to endure mama through her illness. I am grateful that I could hold her beautiful hands each night and feed her words, even if it took her 30 minutes to complete just one sentence. I am grateful that even when she couldn't say anything back, she could look at me with those pretty eyes and smile back at me, knowing that I was there for her in the moments when she couldn't be there for herself. I am grateful that her words—even with aid—continue to reap blessings in my life, today. That's the true work of a mama's prayer.

Amen.

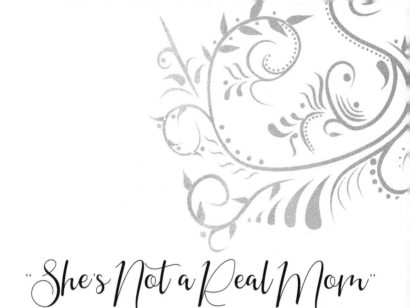

"She's Not a Real Mom"

I WAS BORN AND MOSTLY RAISED IN SOUTHERN, sunny California. Although I did experience a lot of racism, I surprisingly had a space of empathy when it came to mama's disability. My friends and their family did not take it as being too weird or strange, but I also didn't introduce many people to her or the idea of her. Some would ask why I would often talk about daddy and doing things with him instead of talking about mama, but it was because I didn't have the opportunities to do things with her. If and when I did do things with mama, a lot of people probably wouldn't understand it in the context that I would describe it. Therefore, if people hung out with me after school, they would often experience daddy or grandpa because that is who I spent most of my time with, and what would make most sense to them. On top of this, my grandpa was white, so it added an extra layer of complexity in explaining to others my very unique family dynamic.

In the middle of my childhood, my family and I decided to relocate to Elizabeth City, North Carolina. It definitely was a cultural shock as I went from a majority white school to a majority black school. Nonetheless, I was initially excited about this because I endured extensive bullying at school for being "too dark" to play with the other kids. I remember going home to daddy and asking him why didn't I have light skin like mama. As a five-year old I had no full understanding that race was such a problem since there were so many different skin tones in my immediate and extended family. Nonetheless, daddy was not afraid to explain the ins and outs of racism and how every single person in this family will have a different experience with law enforcement and authority. After dealing with it for a few more days, I came home, ran a bath of water, and poured a half of container of Clorox bleach in the tub. I was going to find some way to become as fair skinned as mama so that I would stop getting picked on at school. Daddy must have smelled the odd bleach smell and came in the nick of time before I stepped into the tub. He was stunned, surprised, and a little saddened. "Why would you think to do this!?" he asked, holding back hints of fear. "I just want my skin to look like mama's. This girl at school keeps telling me that I am too dark to play with her and that I look like the concrete, and everyone talks about how pretty mama is, so if she's pretty, I want to look like her." It was such a weird dichotomy at the time because everyone knew that I did look just like daddy as a kid but I also highly resembled mama. Daddy comforted me as he drained the bathtub, and let's just say that in about four days, that girl no longer had anything to say to me about my skin or my looks. Daddy knew how to make things go away for both mama and I. So, I think the point has been made as to why I was so excited to move to a mostly black school.

Being a young girl living in the south came with a lot of environmental norms that I was not aware of when I lived in California. Living in the small city of North Carolina, having a functional mother in the house was expectedly essential. Therefore, when everyone would see daddy pick me up from school daily, the other kids would always ask, "where's your mama?" When I would share with my friends (or so-called friends) the condition of mama, it was nearly impossible for them to understand. I remember after describing my mama to one of my classmates, they turned their head sideways and stated,

"So basically, you don't have a real mom."

Cindy Rae was easily the most beautiful woman I had ever seen in my life, and I only knew her through her disability so that says a lot. While being in a far progression of her MS, she had a 10 lb baby girl —natural birth. I have never seen a day that she wasn't shining her beautiful smile. I remember the times when she would use the small cognitive energy that she had to muster, "I love you" to me. She fought strongly through each day as the beautiful mama that she was. She was the most powerful and the most real mama that could ever exist, in my eyes. She was a human being who breathed, ate, slept, and did other things just like every other human. She laughed, cried, smiled, and frowned just like anyone who has emotions. So, to hear that others thought mama wasn't real was completely absurd.

But, sometimes, that thought would seep in.

I remember two specific times when I invited my friends over to hang out. When the first friend came over, I was so excited yet so nervous on how they may receive mama.

When they rang the doorbell, I quickly rushed to mama's room and slowly closed her door with a sigh of grief upon my face, looking at her through the waning crack. I didn't want to demonstrate that I was ashamed of her, but I didn't know how to handle someone possibly not accepting her for who she was. I then hustled to the door and brought my friend in. She wanted a tour of the house so I of course showed her around. When we approached mama's door, my heart began to increasingly accelerate. "Whose room is that?" my friend asks. I mentioned that it's mama's room but she's not allowed to see her. She was so confused as to why she couldn't so I just decided to rip the band-aid off and swung open the door. There mama was, in her motorized hospital bed, watching TV in peace. My friend softly said "oh, I didn't know…" and became very silent. Without understanding what I did at the time, I then chose to project upon her silence that she felt shame or awkwardness towards seeing a person in such a state. I then felt slightly ashamed. Mostly, I felt guilty that I exposed her to something that maybe she couldn't handle or that would traumatize her. I quickly closed the door back, and diverted us into going outside and playing. I always made sure that when she came over, we would just go outside and play the entire time to avoid the space of this pain for the future. She never brought up mama ever since.

The second friend was really excited about finally coming to hang out with me at my nice house. My daddy always liked to talk to the parents of my friends to ensure that he knows them and that they know his intentions while having their child in his care. So, daddy calls her mom to become acquainted. During the call he walks into another room as his countenance lowers. I sneak down the hall to listen, but I didn't want to go too far and get caught listening so that I would ruin the entire Operation: "Have Friend Come Over". When daddy got off the call, he walked back down the hallways and I scurried back to my original post in my room. Daddy then forwardly told me that this friend isn't coming over anymore. I was so confused and assumed that maybe daddy just didn't like something that the mom said and so I left it at that. The next day I went to school and saw my friend that I invited over before class. I giddily went to go say "hey girl!" and she returned with a lack-luster "hey". I was slightly thrown off and then remembered that somehow our plans changed about her coming over. Daddy must have said no, so she must be upset. I thought to bring up why she wasn't allowed to come over, and at first she did not want to tell me. After extensively prying, I found out that after daddy told her mom about our household, they thought that since mama was disabled, then it is not a safe house with my daddy as the only functioning adult. My heart plunged, my limbs were cold, and I was pale. She couldn't make eye contact with me as she decided to walk away, ending the conversation. I felt my heart struggling to continue beating as tears welled into my eyes. I blinked them away but they couldn't stop flowing. I did not realize this until adulthood, but I internalized this as shame. I was ashamed of mama. Maybe they were right—maybe I didn't have a real mom.

The topic quickly circulated around the school as people began to identify me as the one with the slow mom, or disabled mom, or no mom. It didn't help that I didn't understand what MS was, so I couldn't even describe it to people. Since everyone knew what cancer was, I just said that she had really bad cancer. I felt so isolated not being able to open up to others on who mama really was. Even when I finally found a couple of friends who weren't afraid to say hello to her or be near her, I was already stained by the shame that others imprinted in me, so I assumed in my head that they were judging her. I now call this vicarious social anxiety, or social liability (none of these are real terms, but they work for me). Essentially, from the situations with mama, I learned to be anxious based on how an external person feels about a person associated with me, not necessarily me. I saw mama as a social liability because who she was made others feel uncomfortable or awkward. Additionally, it always made me feel confused because I wanted them to see how amazing she is to me, but all they have the capacity to see is everything that was wrong with her.

From that moment with my friend, everything changed. I went home that day and I hid all of the pictures of her post-diagnosis from my room. I recognized that the normal life that I adapted was not normal to anyone except daddy and I. Were we living in a lie? I then told daddy what my friend at school said and asked why he didn't tell me. He mentioned that he didn't want to hurt my feelings or mama's feelings on how the world views her. I just didn't get it—why could no one else see what we saw? Why wasn't she enough to be considered as a full parent? Why do we ignore the "ability" part in "disability"?

Because of this, I made a strong commitment to protect us so that this kind of pain would never happen again. I didn't really allow people to come to my house until she was moved into the nursing home. If she was home, I would just avoid anyone going in her room, even if it was right across the hall. I couldn't process what my life truly meant now that I was exposed to hurtful and hateful opinions that mama was less of a mama than the others simply because of her health. In the midst of this internal turmoil, I started to pull away from mama. I let their thoughts win. How can the most beautiful woman I know who brought me into the world at 10 pounds become so invisible to me?

As I continued to grow as a person, I had to convict myself on these thoughts to heal from my mama pains. Deep down inside, I knew I had an absolutely real mama, and I truly knew that she was a superhero. She was incredible. Did I mention that she was a very real mama? She had real traumas and real wounds. Real emotions when she heard my friends' awkward comments about her from outside the room. She had real pleasures and joys. Real smiles when she saw her daughter come in the room and spend time with her. She defined mama beyond the true definition, yet not easily defined by the common eye. You had to experience her motherhood from within. She taught me more about being a woman without speaking a word than most women did throughout my life. She loved me more than everyone in the world. The lack of experience, fear, and discomfort of others somehow took precedence over my own truths that I genuinely experienced, firsthand. That was a battle that was hard to shake, but definitely worth shaking to truly understand, experience, and believe who mama really was.

I reminded myself to pray for those who wrestle with having a disabled parent and battling against the worldly views, because we are truly taught to see flaws over ability. It scared me to know that sometimes that's all my friends would ever see and feel bad for me. But I didn't see it as a loss at all—I had the best mama in the school. I pray daily that the love I have for my mama pressed through to her heart a lot further than the vicarious insecurity of others I carried. With most of the world not believing in her, I know she needed her daughter to. I pray that my mama always knew that even when the world couldn't see it, I could always see that she was the best, most beautiful and most fulfilling mama.

She was definitely a real mama.

Eww, Mama Drools

AS IF THERE AREN'T ENOUGH THINGS THAT MAKE this disability hard to manage, there are also some factors that may come in as aesthetically displeasing both for the person involved and the surrounding parties. MS can create quite diverse body responses depending on the severity and on the stage the person is currently in. One symptom that may come as displeasing to most is that because of the delayed or damaged messages reaching certain body parts (or all), there are certain muscles that cannot be controlled in a reasonable time. As a result, mama was not able to control the muscles in her face as well, specifically with salivating. She would often aspirate on food because she was not able to chew well, or it would just fall out of her mouth. We would always be sure to keep a nice towel by her mouth so her shirts do not become ruined from food when she could not control it. Other times, she would just randomly drool because her body didn't signal her mouth and throat to swallow. This was the most difficult to take in as a child, for it pained me that she could not fully indulge in the simplest joys of eating or to enjoy life without worrying about drools accidentally coming out of your mouth. It was also difficult to take in because there was always such a negative connotation towards those who had a disability that caused them to drool. As I saw so many people be made fun of both at school and on television for their developmental disability, it was so hard to recognize that mama would have been the punchline to their jokes.

Mama's drooling would be sporadic so it was almost an Olympic game to catch. This was especially present during family pictures. Every single time we would have mama dolled up and pretty with the most decorated shirt that we can find. Then, right before the flash, her face muscles would give out. Daddy and I would quickly grab a towel to clean her and sit her face up. I could tell that it was slightly irritating and exhausting to anyone who wasn't consistently used to it like we were, but I think it truly taught us patience and learning how to enjoy mama just as she was, not how she could be that would make life easier. There would be times when company comes to visit us and she would accidentally and randomly drool around them. We always felt in a scurry to explain to others what was so normal and common for ourselves. The easiest thing for us to was to keep her head elevated at just the perfect place where she wasn't sitting too far forward that it would force her to drool, but also not too far back that she could possibly choke. Again—an Olympic sport. But it was fun always keeping mama clean and making sure that she feels beautiful. Although she was disabled, she was human. So, we wanted to make sure that we still treated her as such and didn't just leave her in a state as if she's forgotten about in any way.

Daddy and I also made sure to watch what we said around mama, as well as what she watched. Because there was so much content on television directly towards making fun of people who were physically disabled, we made sure that we would quickly cut that off around mama. We didn't want to perpetuate any reminders of her disability, nor indulge in anything that makes fun of the very true circumstances that were right in our household. Although we did everything we could to protect such narratives, it often seeped through for us because it was an assured way to deal with our reality. As a young kid, I was still navigating how to make the most of this situation while still respecting mama. Sometimes the jokes seemed funny, but I recognized that I had the privilege of not knowing how it feels to be the actual recipient of the jokes. Even though it was my mama, I had to make an extended effort to understand how this directly impacts her.

I recall a time around the age of five where my thoughts came into reality on how I felt about mama's motor skills. Daddy was wrapping up one of his great meals and brought it in the bedroom for us to eat. After ending our daily prayers, we got ready to dig into our plates. Daddy usually feeds mama first so that she doesn't miss out on us eating together. Daddy then realized that he needed to grab something from the kitchen and asked me to quickly start feeding mama. I looked at him with disgust and said aloud, "eww, she drools!" With a wrath of disappointment and pain, daddy scurried down the hallway to me and gently nudged me to step into the hallway and away from my mama. As a five-year old without a filter, I wasn't sure what caused such fury in daddy but I scurried along to find out.

He briskly asked, "why would you say that in front of her?" Confused on his obvious question, he then continued with a follow-up explanation. "Do you understand that mama has a disease? There are things her body will do that may not seem normal to everyone else or even us. But, we have to make it normal to us because she IS normal to us. She's your mama. Imagine how she feels hearing you think that she is gross."

With no fault to daddy, I felt like the lowest person in the world. He was right—I did wonder how that made her feel hearing me say that with such conviction and pure disgust. I loved my mama so much and I truly loved everything about her, even if I didn't understand it or if I thought it was gross. I loved everything about her. I couldn't imagine hearing my daughter saying that I was gross, and I don't think I would ever want to find out. I couldn't imagine watching my daughter stand distantly from the bed because she didn't understand me, grossed out, which is exactly what I did at that moment. I could just imagine the subconscious expression of disgust upon my face that mama had to see from her very own offspring. Nonetheless, the beautiful thing about that moment with mama is that when I commented on her drooling right in front of her face, she then just looked at me and smiled. Such a motherly love—that perhaps in the midst of embarrassment, sadness, or pain, she made sure to bring joy, comfort, and understanding to her only offspring. I honestly felt even worse after that.

I told daddy I was so sorry for saying something that could possibly hurt mama and that I would go in to apologize to her and feed her. He thanked me. Although I was willing to go back in the room and feed her, I had not still fully comprehended what this meant on how I felt about mama drooling. I still thought it was gross. And, I still thought it was beautiful. I was anxiously nervous, but I knew that I needed to pull it together and show mama I do love her—while she's drooling. I slowly crept back towards the bedroom and peaked my head around the door frame. I just looked at her, watching TV as she waited for the opportunity to eat. I know that she has to be hungry. I slowly walked in, and reached onto the towel to pick up her bowl of crab salad from our eating towel and grabbed the spoon nearby. I slowly opened the container and laid the top upon the bed. I then took the spoon and I swirled it around a few times to make sure that the ingredients were mixed well, and also to stall towards the moment where I would have to feed her and look her in the eyes after saying something so hurtful. I felt my heart begin to thumb in my chest and my quite hunger-struck stomach become uneasy as I listened to the moist mixtures of the salad tossing around in anticipation. I rubbed my sweaty fingers together from stirring so much, and finally took a scoop into the crab salad to put on the spoon. I slowly looked up at mama, and stared for a short second hoping that the salad wouldn't fall off the spoon in my personal moment of conviction. "Open up ma," I said in the faintest voice and the greatest anticipation. She wiggled to slightly turn her head towards me and forced her mouth open as wide as she could. I slid the spoon into her mouth and she bit down to close. I slid the spoon out and gently wiped her mouth with the towel underneath her chin. "I'm sorry mama for what I said. I don't think you're gross." I forced myself to then watch her eat, as she sometimes chewed and sometimes took a break. Some of the food would fall from her mouth, and some she swallowed. She stared at the television while chewing and then turned her large brown eyes towards me. It's like she could see into my soul. She looked so innocent. I can only imagine how hard she tries to just enjoy all of her food every time she eats. Her strength and resilience in these moments truly inspired me, and I saw it the most when she looked at me. I then wiped her mouth again of the spilled food, and then smiled at her. She smiled back at me.

Over the years it stopped bothering me that mama drooled. Most of the time, I barely noticed. I learned that the idea of it being gross came from others and not really from my own perspective. Honestly, daddy and I saw it as a normal human function just like anything else. I learned that often we put disgust on things that we are afraid to deeply understand or that we are not comfortable with. I learned that it was vulnerable to embrace mama drooling because that required me to accept her at her rawest form. Specifically in black families, it is not very common for people to fully open themselves to others in a raw, unapologetic, unmasked state. We are taught that isn't proper, or that "everyone doesn't want to know/see all of that". It became so normal for me to see family and close people only show the parts of themselves that are favorable that when I see someone give all of themselves, it feels so awkward that my brain registers it as disgust. With mama, she had no other choice but to do so because she did not have the motor or cognitive skills to hide anything. This was a unique demonstration of love and connection that she could not control but we had the opportunity to receive and embrace. Imagine if all of us gave our 100% selves to someone else—our family, kids, siblings, spouse, friends, or whoever. How much different would our lives be? How whole would we feel? This is why it initially felt awkward to receive mama's drooling. Not because it was gross, but because it was a vulnerable love that was different from any other experience of love. She was giving all of herself to me. And, I was learning that I deserved to receive it. It has now impacted on why I am so open and transparent to others. If you can't receive who I fully am, then what's the point of receiving just a part of me?

Over time, I had to create a space of forgiveness for a five-year old girl with very little development of emotional intelligence to finally connect with mama as I wished. It wasn't the easiest thing to process right away for a young girl yet I did want to figure it out so that I could love mama the way that she deserved. I thank daddy for quickly having a transparent conversation with me about our truest reality with mama. The conversation with daddy reminded me that her physical responses never deterred who she truly was. She still was a human being with real human responses. She still had real feelings and emotions. And, she was hungry and ready to eat! Although many sectors taught us to devalue people who didn't have a similar ability level to us, I learned to look at people past face value and celebrate what is within, starting with mama. The world may still see her with a disability or disabled, but I saw mama with all ability or all-able.

Mama's Sunshine

1 F YOU KNEW MAMA, THEN YOU DEFINITELY KNEW of her smile. Whether you met her in one short encounter or if you knew her for a lifetime, mama's smile truly transformed lives. Mama had a beautiful, bright, and perfect smile. Physically, she had sparkling white and perfectly aligned teeth that would shine in all of the most radiant spaces. Of all the things we did for mama, we always made sure to take special care of her beautiful teeth. Every morning and night we would grab the pink bowl from the bathroom, grab her electric toothbrush with the red band, and a fresh mini pouch of Colgate toothpaste, and a cup of hot water, and brushed her teeth in her bed. Just along with her hair, I loved seeing the radiance of her smile in the midst of everything going on. Knowing that we could help perfect mama's smile each day not only gave joy to her, but her smile also gave a radiance to daddy and I.

MS definitely has a strong impact on the abilities of the muscles within the face. It can cause jaw pain, muscle spasms, and as strongly and previously covered, drooling. MS can also cause a decrease or strain in facial expression. Therefore, it was a literal blessing to see how much mama smiled. She smiled all of the time, even if no one was watching. And, this wasn't just a smile that brought joy upon your face. Mama had a beautiful and inspiring way of smiling through her spirit. Every single time I saw mama (until her face was not able to move much anymore) she had a smile on her face. She would even sometimes strain her muscles a little to make sure that she smiled. Oftentimes, daddy and I would ask her to smile just for the beauty of it, and she would right on the spot. What a beautiful smile. It was so beautiful because it came from a genuine place inward. I mean, how could someone who was paralyzed in a bed in her late twenties and into her thirties be able to smile at every given moment? Mama taught me the very subtle but vast difference between happiness and joy, and it was definitely a lesson that carried with me throughout life.

As a child, I often found any moment I could to put a smile on mama's face. I knew that it was one of the few ways that I could fully connect with her and how we could experience emotion together. I remember a specific moment when I sat down and told mama about my first basketball game during middle school. I was so excited to tell her about this game because I knew it would probably make her smile harder than anyone.

To give context, mama was also a hooper back in her days. She played at Watterson High School in Columbus, Ohio and then played for The Ohio State University until her illness overcame her. Looking over some of her old newspaper clippings and her stat book, we had a lot in common on how we played. We both played so, it felt as the highest honor to let her know how hard I played. Although mama was much taller at 5'10, we both had pretty beastly stats around rebounds and points. Knowing that this piece of her still resonates within me felt as the highest connection to her and felt as if I continued her legacy. My grandma, grandpa, and daddy all attended this game, and they all agreed that I played just like mama, which brought such joy upon us all.

I assertively anticipated the drive home and the opportunity to burst into the house and tell mama what happened before dinner and prayers could even begin. When daddy pulled into the garage and parked the car, I was excited to take off. I jolted from the car, and ran in the doors yelling, "MA!" before anything else could happen or anyone else could get to her. For the lack of physical ability she had, a smile never seemed to be difficult to gleam across her face when she saw me. Exasperated in breath, I walked beside her bed, held onto her side rail to prop up my body, and I began to tell every detail of the greatest highlights from such a monumental game. Daddy saw that this was a moment of quality time so he headed to the kitchen. I started with telling mama I played post today, which meant that this was the position where we were often near the bucket to rebound, score in the paint, or to block someone's shot. Mama played post as well so I know this made her excited. I told her that I had 15 points and 7 rebounds, a high number of rebounds for someone my height at the time. I went on and on about the number of rebounds I had and how fun it was to be strong enough to block people out from the basket so I could get the shot. Mama continued to nod and increasingly smile as I told the story, which were even greater motor skills that I've seen in her yet. I then told her about this one incredible fade-away shot that I swished in my defender's face. "Mama! They passed me the ball in the corner, and you know that's my favorite shot. I took a couple of quick dribbles, picked the ball up quickly, faded back and hit the shot—nothing but net. The crowd went so crazy!" Mama exclaimed a small moan, which was her communication of excitement at the furthest extent. Initially, I had the expectancy that she would not say anything back, as I knew her speech at this point was strongly decreasing. But, to my surprise, mama gleamed a smile from ear to ear and moaned away in so much excitement that her baby girl played so great, just as she did. Seeing all 32 of her teeth shining on my excitement ceased the incredible moment beyond my athletic abilities. I honestly wanted to keep playing well so I could come home and tell her about it.

I can never erase after that first basketball game how it felt to ride all the way home in excitement to make mama smile. It was my motivation and I came to believe that it was her therapy. It was our way to connect in an astronomical way beyond my greatest imagination. Before every game, I thought about her. I thought about how I needed to play to make her smile. I even thought about her before my academic performances, talent shows, speeches, and award ceremonies. I had to make her proud. I couldn't wait to go home and tell her so I could see her smile. When I saw her smile, my life instantly enhanced. This was the power of her smile. She made you feel capable. She made you feel like you could do anything. She made you feel valuable—just from her smile.

Someone else that deeply enjoyed mama's smile was daddy. My daddy is a very sweet man but also a tough man. While he was tender as can be, you wouldn't catch daddy smiling with all of his teeth too many times—except when he was with mama. The way that mama made my daddy smile with her smile was incredibly magical and breathtaking. You can't even make this type of love story up on how two people could keep each other alive (literally, keep each other alive) without barely saying words or fully touching bodies. Daddy would always come in the house to kiss on mama's face and then mess with her playfully as she giggled. Mama couldn't fully laugh over the years but she definitely giggled and shared small laughs resounding as stretched moans mixed with overextended smiles. When daddy messed with her, it was always there. He would always say, "there's my Cindy Lou from the Caribou" and she would always giggle away and blush. Even when I was in the greatest of trouble, mama would sometimes smile at my daddy in hopes of curving his discipline. My daddy would jokingly come to mama's bed saying, "now girl, don't try to use that pretty smile to get April B out of trouble. I know what you are doing with that pretty smile!" They would then chuckle together at each other and he would gently tickle her as they would boldly smile together. It was truly incredible, and relieving, how mama's smile could turn some of the hardest times into some of the best times for daddy and I. I prayed for love like that for the rest of the years of my life. Her smile reflected security. She felt safe with daddy. She felt loved. And, I'm sure she felt lucky that as handsome as daddy was, he picked her to spend the rest of his life with (well, honestly, as beautiful as mama was, I think he was really the lucky one). Nonetheless, mama's smile was the greatest enrichment of love in the house because it represented so much more than happiness. The significant irony that a person who is disabled is the greatest vessel of joy in our house is the greatest demonstration of God's truest work.

Picture days with mama would be fun—not just because of the drooling—but because it was exciting to see the beauty of mama in a snapshot. Pictures of mama always excited me because she was absolutely gorgeous and I loved capturing it for others so they wouldn't just see her disability. Mama would always make the picture so much brighter with her kind eyes partnered with her million-dollar smile. Anytime that she saw a camera, she knew that it was an opportunity to make it shine. I often look back upon those pictures and reflect on the power of her happiness. As I am looking at a picture of a disabled woman, I also see a huge smile as if nothing else is even happening. She looks joyful. She looks free. She looks hopeful. The power in her smile often reminded me that I could believe in joy, freedom, and hope too.

As I became older, I would often think of mama's smile as a symbol of resilience. I often wondered if it was a cover up of her truest pains, or if it was a declaration to find the best in every single day of her circumstances. With either answer, it still amazed me that mama found the strength to smile every single day, consistently—even when no one was looking. When I would get upset or cry over the smallest things, I often wondered, how can I find joy like mama did? How can I find something to smile about when there were so many things that brought so much pain? I would even look forward to coming to see mama after school just because I knew that she would smile when she saw me. I knew that if nothing else had the power to make me smile that day, she would let me borrow hers for the day. A truly undeniable demonstration of love, grace, peace, and joy without having to say a word. Maybe it was the perfection of her teeth, or the pronounced high cheek bones that rose above her eye creases, or how it was the easiest movement that she could successfully perform. Maybe it was also knowing that in the midst of any barrier, she has found strength to smile. Whatever the reason may be, it has been more than enough to find the biggest smile possible in every single day and to hope that my smile can impact someone else's life, just like mama's did for me. When I smile I see her because I have found a way to adapt her smile—internally and externally. I now realize that it was more than a formation of her countenance, but that it was an alignment in her heart coming to life.

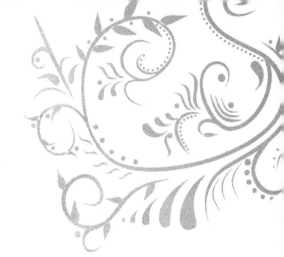

Mama, Let's Cry Together

YOU WOULD THINK THAT BEING DISABLED would prohibit mama from sharing intimate moments with me. Contrary to the perceived obvious, mama was truly there for me in the most emotionally critical times. One thing in particular that stood out to me is how she would cry with me when I cried. This would be almost in any scenario, and it would always feel so comforting. Just as bright as her smile was, that is how resonating her tears were. Although a partial reason for her tearful responses is an involuntary symptom of Multiple Sclerosis, it truly served as a very timely and empathetic experience that I got to share with mama.

Crying spells are a common symptom of MS. It has something to do with a hormonal and cognitive response that sometimes misfires at random times. Therefore, my mama would cry at times, but she wasn't necessarily sad all of those times. It was often hard to navigate how to comfort her when I never knew if she was truly sad or if it was a crying spell, but even so I would make sure to give her attention when I could. It was sometimes frustrating for others because they wouldn't know how to stop it, or confusing because they aren't sure what caused it. But when I would cry on my own, I honestly didn't often think about if mama was having a crying spell or if she was actually crying with me. Even with her sporadic instances of tears, I was assured that she really did cry with me, as the timing was quite impeccable. I can still hear the bellowing moans of her voice as tears streamed down our face, in matching tone, serendipitously. In those moments it made me cry more because I felt safe to cry. Sometimes, it also made me cry less because I knew that someone understood how I felt and it brought me more relief. In both ways, it always felt comforting to not cry alone.

Crying was also quite vulnerable for me. Although I lived in quite a comforting home, it was also patterned by normalized cultural practices of shrinking emotional response or expression. Although this wasn't intentionally malicious, at a young age I taught myself that I need to be cautious on how I express emotions, specifically crying, so that I do not cause anyone else to feel uncomfortable or so that I wouldn't come off as a nuisance. Over time, it bred the common narrative of being the "strong black girl" while being broken and fragile within. Knowing this often left me with numerous unresolved pains as a child. Luckily, it wasn't the heaviest of pains, but there were certainly enough accumulated pains to create a pattern of silence. Even through such a wall of emotional security, I knew how important and comforting mama's presence was when she would experience emotions with me. We commonly use the phrase, "a mama's touch", but her touch was touchless, wordless, and without movement. To know that she didn't have to tell me any cliche phrases, or any rehearsed gestures of comfort, or hand me food in hopes of lightening my mood—just her existence was the greatest of emotional safety.

A particular moment that mama always cried with me is when I got in trouble with daddy, which wasn't too often, but it was enough to take note. Daddy was loving but firm in ensuring that I would become a well-behaved child without being a nuisance to the greater world. As the true disciplinarian that he was, daddy would make it clear when I crossed the behavioral boundaries that he set and would often have some form of reprehension, often with me resulting to tears. I was quite sensitive about hurting others, so even the smallest look would break my fragile dams and the tears would flood. Sometimes, if it was serious enough, I would break down pretty badly. In a matching tandem, mama then bellows in tears along with me. She would stare distantly with trickling tears falling from face and gently moaning along. I had a lot of shame around crying, so to know that mama offered such an innocent experience of crying with me, it truly meant the world. A beautiful thing that always comforted me in this moment is when my mama would cry with me. I felt as if my pain did not go unnoticed.

I knew this somehow had to irritate daddy that there were now two people crying in a moment that he is trying to redirect behavior, but I saw it as my saving grace. Even with such, daddy he often mentioned how special it was that she would cry with me. A woman who is completely disabled was still able to emotionally comfort me—that is truly one of a kind gift that no disability could impact. Mama truly made sure that I never felt alone. Although I had two present parents in my life, there was something special about the emotional presence of mama, even when she wasn't saying a word.

Mama and daddy both knew that I wasn't the biggest fan of our family pictures. For some reason, it annoyed me and stressed me out, but I honestly wasn't sure why. We would put so much effort into family pictures by matching our colors and patterns, bringing out our best hair styles, and making sure that we looked top notch at all times. Despite our greatest efforts, I would always find some way to ruin them. During our first shoot, the best shot was a picture of daddy holding me on his shoulder as I was softly trickling tears from completely breaking down right before. Everyone still looked picture perfect, and mama's bright and beautiful smile was right in the middle. The second picture day was the most memorable of them all. We were already slightly frantic and running late to our appointment at the studio. As we got everyone packed up in the cars, and secured mama as well, we headed out. When we arrived at the studio, we quickly got set up and in place, but I just wasn't feeling it. So of course again, I cried. It was very unpleasant timing but I truly hated family pictures. Daddy tried to firmly direct my attitude but it wasn't really settling in, so I cried more. Seeing that I really felt a lot of discomfort and no one to really give me comfort, mama started crying as well. You could then probably place eggs on the top of everyone's head and make a breakfast platter because there was so much frustration in the studio. Because neither of us could really be "calmed down", the pictures began! There are actual photographs of mama and I crying in the picture while I'm holding a little toy. We looked great, just with tears. Luckily there were other pictures of the family without my wild crying antics (they removed me from the photo), and of course, there was the classic photo of daddy holding me on his shoulder as I'm softly sobbing. Although there was tons of frustration during family photos, having mama cry with me made me feel so supported in spaces where I thought I would feel alone.

Mama would also cry with me while watching sad TV shows or movies. As a family, we loved the opportunity to watch things that would pull at our heart strings. We would watch shows like All in The Family, Andy Griffith, Good Times, and other old shows that highlighted authentic experiences in the lives of those around us. We also loved watching movies that had an emotional plot that we could all connect to. Some of our favorites included Philadelphia, Cast

Away, John Q, and Radio. As we sat around the TV watching a movie, it would be so comforting to look over with my teary eyes and see mama trickling tears as well. While there are so many rationales on how media and entertainment can be harmful, it can also bring us as a family together and experience emotions that we may have not been able to encounter in a normal setting. I was often thankful for movies and TV shows that allowed an opportunity for us to create emotion together as a family since there were very limited things that mama could do. I can imagine it was also special to mama that we are both so tender-hearted that we enjoy crying together about similar things.

I didn't have any siblings growing up. So, I missed out on the experience that people had of looking to their brother or sister to find emotional comfort and connection. This was hard because I witnessed a lot growing up that I wished I had someone else in the house to validate that I was not crazy for how I felt. Nonetheless, the presence of mama's emotions came as a ram in the bush, as it made me feel like I didn't grow up on my own. I knew there were spaces that perhaps she wished she could do more, but to know that she could lend her emotions to me in a time where she cognitively and physically could not give much more gave all of the strength I needed to survive and thrive through really hard situations. Mama's tears softened everything. She made me feel okay.

Mama's cry was always so comforting, yet I also could tell that she was finding ways to release the pain that she may have not been able to express in other spaces. I often wondered as a young girl how it felt to know that mama had the opportunity to cry along with her daughter. I also wondered if she cried when I wasn't there, and if she did, what would make her cry? Did my expression of tears make her feel as if she didn't have to cry alone anymore? I felt our heaviness run through the rivers together, free-flowing into the lands of liberation and bliss. It was only pure serendipity and alignment that mama's crying spells somehow matched up with my tearful moments. Even in our lowest of times, there was a cleansing security of peace, experienced in togetherness.

Mama had such a powerful presence of emotional expression that I often enjoyed the opportunity to exist in her presence. There were times where I would come home, silently walk to her room, and sit beside her bed. She would often have her television on TV Land, low volumed and bright screened. I would occasionally put my hand on hers and just feel her presence. As a daughter, I wish that I gave a lot more energy towards sharing quality time with her, but I was continuing to process what it truly meant to have this unique experience of daughterhood. Even if daddy was there, I would find the space to connect intimately with my mama. Having those experiences of crying with mama subconsciously created a deep and intimate connection that I would come to miss dearly when mama went to the nursing home. I recognized that when she had to go, I never got any more moments with just her and I alone. When we visited, it was always daddy and I. Even in the smallest moments when it was just me and her, mama's impact was so bold and grace-filled.

Presently, many people do ask why I choose to go through things without telling anyone or choose to withhold showing emotion. Through mama, I learned that true empathy does not have to come from any strenuous action. For someone who was completely disabled to make me feel safe to be vulnerable shows that love and support is a basic human gesture—we just have to be willing to tap into it. I struggled to find anyone whose love and support compared to mama, yet I also knew that a love like hers was rare to find. I had to learn over the years how to find emotional security, even if she is not physically present. I do have someone who will always cry with me, and who will always feel my pain. My mama always reminded me that I am loved, forgiven, and that I am not alone. And, I hope that she always felt the same from me in return.

Mama's Strawberry Cake

AMONGST ALL THE BEAUTIFUL THINGS ABOUT mama, she had thirty-two beautiful and shining teeth. With this, there was a 33rd tooth that served her well upon her mouth—mama had a sweet tooth. Mama loved her sweets, cakes, pies, and candies. It was quite fitting as daddy and I both love to indulge in yummy desserts. We enjoyed the opportunity to bake something special on the weekends, allow the aroma of sweet pastries to sweep the air composition, and have something tasty for mama to taste and for us all to deeply enjoy. Of all the delicious sweets we made, mama's favorite of them all was strawberry cake. Oh, how my mama loved a fresh strawberry cake, especially with real strawberries. It was such a treat to not only indulge into such a wonderful delicacy, but to also experience through such a fun cooking adventure with daddy!

Daddy was an incredible cook and baker. He brought me into the kitchen at a very young age and taught me secret tips to pass along one day to my own family someday. I was always quite excited to help with any of our meals, but there was a unique excitement about making something especially for mama. I loved the special opportunity for her to taste the love that I am personally giving to her and wanted to make sure that the food represents exactly how much I love her. When I made strawberry cake for mama, I wanted to make sure that all of the warm, gooey happiness that she enjoys comes from my little brown hands and into the specific composition of the batter.

With MS being so severe for her, it truly was a privileged honor for her to enjoy food as much as possible and ensure that we give her the best things that she could eat. There were some foods that she couldn't fully chew or swallow, steak for example. So, daddy and I always made sure that whatever we made mama could be manageable for her but also taste incredible so that she doesn't feel as if she is missing anything. When we made strawberry cake for mama, or any sweet for her, it seemed extra special because I know how sweets make me feel. It is a piece of life that she can enjoy and can probably escape from anything else that is going on in her life for that one brief bite. Although I didn't like strawberry cake at all when I first tried it, I grew to appreciate it over the years because it was specially made for mama.

I can never forget the rich smell of fresh California strawberries filling my nose as daddy and I pulled the ingredients out and prepared to cook strawberry cake for us all to enjoy. We found all of the mixing bowls and cooking utensils and pulled out the rest of the ingredients. Daddy and I then blended spices of sugars, extracts, flours, and strawberry flavors. We cracked the eggs and whisked the milk. We made messes that we were excited to clean up again soon. We bellowed laughter of joy throughout the residential hallways as the aromas of the sweet, delectable joys wrapped around our bodies. During the entire time, the spread of my biggest smile never left my face because I knew that I was making something that would bring joy to mama.

After the baking process was complete, we would add the final whipped icing to cover the warm cake. The over-intoxicating scent waters my eyes and salivates my taste buds in excitement. I secretly take a quick lick of icing and relish in the pure satisfaction of successful baking. We let it set aside as we first decided to have dinner. I scurry to set up our eating area, as I do not want to show any time wasted in getting to our delectable masterpiece. We then sit beside mama to say our prayers. Throughout the evening prayers, all I can honestly think about are strawberry cakes, and cakes of strawberries. After the final amen, I quickly dive into our dinner. I hoped that maybe if I eat dinner faster, I will have the opportunity to get to the strawberry cake quicker. Of course this plan never worked, so I waited patiently and eagerly after scarfing down my dinner. I would watch daddy feeding mama, taking bite by bite, giggling in between each spill. It was the greatest anticipation towards what amazing reward was to come next. After finally completing her meal, I would work extensively to clear out our eating area, take the dishes into the kitchen, and wait patiently beside the strawberry cake. With a gleaming grin upon my face and a mildly reserved excitement, Daddy gathered the supplies and dishes to prepare in cutting the cake that we worked on so intentionally. Daddy would cut two square pieces for the each of us and put it in a heavy, white bowl. He would then put two scoops of ice cream in each bowl and allow it to slowly melt besides the warm cake. The combination of scents drew a peaceful joy, and little did I know that this sensory experience—the feeling of the cold bowl, the sight of vanilla ice cream pooling around the island of a warm strawberry cake, the incredible scents—all would lodge into my brain as a sign of comfort for the continuance of my life. This would always represent happiness.

We brought mama some cake to her room. I quickly took a bite of my piece as soon as I sat for I could not wait another second to taste such goodness. I gleaned another huge smile as the taste of vanilla slowly hugged the moist, warm, cake. With a mouth full of food, I put my bowl down to tune into mama's response. Daddy fed her the first bite—a small bite so that it was easier to manage. She chewed slowly, and slowly began to smile as she ate. I was so excited. This moment felt as successful as burning a 10-song CD, putting it in your CD player, and seeing if songs actually play. The process was always worth it. It made mama happy.

When it was mama's birthday, daddy and I would always go all out. We would find mama a cute shirt and put it on her. I would find a way to do her hair in a way that is different from all of the other days to ensure that I make her feel incredibly beautiful. Daddy would get her a fun birthday hat and put the string around her neck so that it could securely place upon her head. He would place it on one side of her head so that it had some swag with her birthday style. Daddy and I would spend the day putting together her cake, laced up with clumsy calligraphy of birthday wishes and candles all around. Before bringing mama her cake, we would make sure that it was well lit and presentable. After striking the match and completing the daunting task of successfully lighting every candle, we slowly glided down the hallways, beginning the infamous birthday song.

"Happy birthday to you,
Happy birthday to you,
Happy birthday Cindy Rae-e-e-e-e,
Happy birthday to you!"

Mama would smile and slightly move her head around to the tune as much as she could. I would hold the cake so daddy could grab the camcorder and begin taping the entire moment. He would say goofy but loving things to mama and give her tons of wet kisses. I would then place the cake in front of her face, and let her make a wish. After about 10 seconds, the three of us blew out mama's candles together.

Strawberry cake, although a delectable dessert, served as a staple for a joyful moment within our home. Because it was always made on special occasions for mama, its smell reminded me that things were okay even when it felt like they weren't. When mama was permanently moved to the nursing home, we still made it a point to sneak her in strawberry cake from time to time. The floating aroma of our fresh pastry danced along the hallways and lightened the hearts of each patient, which didn't make us very inconspicuous. It was always the greatest joy to prepare and feed strawberry cake to mama and see how delicious it was to her. There was nothing more meaningful than to know that I could feed her joy. This made such an impact on why I prioritize cooking for others in my continuing years.

There came a time when mama was not able to eat solid foods anymore, which meant that she could no longer eat strawberry cake. Her MS had progressed to a point where she could not fully chew and wallow food without aspiration. This was a hard time for us all because we often bonded heavily over meals. When mama was switched to direct tube feeding into her stomach, daddy and I often thought about the moments we shared in feeding cake and some of her other favorite foods to her. We knew this would probably hurt her, thinking about foods that she wouldn't have the opportunity to taste. Daddy and I talked about this and made a plan that when we would visit her in the nursing home, we wouldn't mention food. We wouldn't mention what we were having for dinner, what I had for lunch at school, or even that I am hungry. We didn't want to remind her of such a big change. The adjustment on her birthday was the hardest because we made sure that no one in the nursing home staff brought up cake. It taught us to celebrate mama in other ways besides just around food.

Blessedly, if we want to experience a slice of mama in our daily routine, we always know what yummy delicacy to turn to. Even in my maturing years, as I bite into a piece of strawberry cake, the feelings of joy and the shine of her smile still resonates within my soul. I often still feel the warm and loving experience of eating strawberry cake and experiencing the exact same joy that I felt the first time we made strawberry cake for mama. It is beautiful how a specific food can ingrain an experience of love, safety, and peace for a lifetime. I hope to not only pass on the recipe to my kids on how to make strawberry cake, but also how to pass along the impact of creating love in the form of art that can bring gladness and joy to someone you deeply love.

It was always a piece of cake.

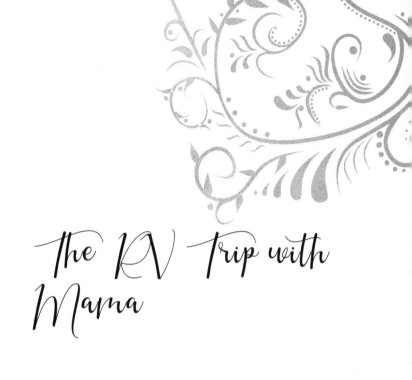

The RV Trip with Mama

$\mathcal{S}$OME OF THE MOST EXCITING MEMORIES FROM my childhood are when we went on family trips. We went all across the nation to different cities and states, exploring new adventures and making new memories. Just to name a few, as a child I've been to the Grand Canyon in Arizona, Mt. Rushmore in South Dakota, Niagara Falls in Canada, Chicago, St. Louis,

Las Vegas, Memphis, Disney world in Florida, Disneyland in California, Atlanta, Charlotte, and quite a few more. We also moved around a lot, so that was a great aid in exploring different spaces of America. As a kid, I was born in San Diego, California, moved briefly to Columbus, Ohio, then briefly to Memphis, TN, then back to San Diego, then to Elizabeth City, NC, and then to Missouri. It was quite an adventure starting new beginnings.

My favorite trips were when we were finally able to take mama on a trip. As her MS symptoms were progressing over the years, it made it a little more difficult to transport her to the vast places we went, so oftentimes she was unfortunately not able to go. Therefore, I was always excited for her to experience everything that we get to experience outside of the household. Even when I saw mama in her outdoor chair or in her wheelchair, it excited me. Mama had a lime green "jerry chair", or geriatric chair, which served as such an exciting pillar of freedom for mama. We would set her chair up by the pool so that she could watch me swim, or on the back patio to get the sun, or in the family room to watch me play games. I sometimes sat in it myself when she wasn't in it to feel mama's warmth or imagine the adventures she could possibly have for the next time we put her in the chair. It was always an exploration to open up the horizons of mama's experiences beyond her motorized bed. My favorite part about moving mama was pulling out her heavy metal lift machine to put her into her chair. Essentially, it had straps that wrapped around mama and it helped us to lift her as we guided around her body. Using this machine was such a signature of hope to me. I got to witness more humanization of mama when she was taken from bed. I used to also love watching daddy lift his wife up and into her chair with effortless strength so that she can relax in a new environment. Honestly, it was a moment of relief that my mama was as human as I thought she was.

Mama was able to fly with us a couple of times during the earlier stages of my childhood as we would go back and forth to Ohio from California to visit daddy's family. It was always exciting to travel as a family unit and allow mama to explore her home city once again in Columbus. We would visit my Big Mama for a warm and loving time, Aunt Bunny and Uncle Brian to laugh and play games, and see my cousins Joe, Ryan, SeRita, and Norman and spend extra quality time of the same warmth and fun. Although mama was fully disabled at the time, it still made for a warming experience for us all.

As mama's MS progressed, we had to look into alternative ways to transport mama for trips. Because of her tubes, rotation she needed, medications, and other things, it made it really difficult to continue in flying mama. Our family decided to move away from San Diego and relocate to a small town in North Carolina. When planning for the move, there were a lot of factors to consider, especially since we were moving across the nation. The most obvious question was then quickly posed as daddy, grandpa and I were passing by each other in the kitchen—

"How do we move mama?"

Since this was a full trip across the country, we realized that we had to get creative with moving mama. This question was quickly resolved in a decision that the most efficient (and fun) way to transport mama was to take an RV trip across the country. We would pack all of the house items to be sent along in a U-Haul, and a few of us would stay back to go in the RV. My grandpa would drive, daddy would take care of mama, and I would play around and help give directions for the trip. It would take about four days if we consistently drove through the entire day. This was probably one of the first and few times that our family would spend so much time together in a very close proximity, so it was exciting to see how this adventure would unfold.

The RV rolled up to the house and I felt my stomach begin to sink realizing that this moment had finally arrived. We were moving to Elizabeth City, North Carolina. My grandma got a new job so it became a new beginning for all of us. Daddy was also going to start his degree in college to get his bachelor's degree. We were really moving away from the life I had known up to this point. Nonetheless, I was able to curb my sinking feelings with the excitement that I got to be in an RV with mama and that we got to travel across the nation together. I snapped back into reality as grandpa hopped out of the RV and asked me to come over and check it out. I can never forget the unique odor of wood and faint sewage covered in aged rose vehicle spray. It was quite spacious and old-fashioned. There was a huge bedroom in the back, a perfect size for mama and all of the few machines and supplies that she needed. There were also a couple of fold out beds that collapsed under the side seats, which is where grandpa and daddy planned to sleep. This meant that I was left to sleep with mama. It was then a realization that I have never had the opportunity to sleep in the bed with mama since I was a baby. Because of how many tubes she had and the sensitivity of her disability, I felt a little afraid to ever sleep with her. Also, mama had a motorized bed that was covered by insurance and given to her. Because of this, no one else was allowed to sleep in the bed except her. It was a really cool bed actually, as it could raise up and down at both the head and feet, and the entire bed could raise up and down as well. It had silver rails on the side so mama wouldn't accidentally slide off one side or the other. All of these cool things, but no one else could ever be in the bed—how unfair. I am not sure who would come to the house and check, but I guess we wanted to maintain the integrity. To make the point, this would truly be a unique opportunity to actually sleep in the same bed as mama, yet this moment built lots of anxiety.

Over the next few days we quickly completed the last of the packing, got mama prepared, put everything in the RV, and got ready to say goodbye to California. I was so excited for all of the activities planned, what we were going to eat, what we were going to watch, what games we were going to play, and what we were going to see along the way. It was bittersweet letting go of this life and risking so much to start somewhere completely new. Despite this, the entire trip was truly unforgettable. There were endless bellows of road songs, ongoing conversations about the truest parts of life, and many outbursts of directions from the nostalgic resource of MapQuest and an atlas. Although it seemed nearly impossible, I made a sure effort to stay awake for every driving moment so that I could indulge in all of the adventure of the long-legged highways. I would sometimes dance back to where mama was lying so I could sing crazy songs to her and open her windows so that she could see the wide-open beauty of our trip and enjoy it together.

The RV also was equipped with a TV set, which was helpful because mama had the TV running throughout the night. Mama would naturally take catnaps throughout the day versus sleeping through the night averagely. Therefore, daddy would always keep the TV on so when she woke up, she had something to entertain her in case we weren't around. Since there was a TV with a VCR player, daddy decided to keep on hand a few tapes to enjoy. On this trip I was introduced to the greatest tunes of the 80's. We had one recorded VCR tape full of music videos from MTV. It started with "Diamonds and Pearls" by Prince, and highlighted songs like "I Do it For You" by Bryan Adams, "Don't Worry, Be Happy" by Bob McFerrin, and "Head to Toe" by Lisa Lisa and the Cult Jam. I remember daddy and I galloping and skipping around the cramped bedroom snapping and whistling along to the bright music video. We would circle mama's bed in our goofy shenanigans singing along to the words,

"Don't worry…be happy!
Don't worry, be happy now—
whoooo-hoo-hoo-hoo-hoo-hoooooooohhh,
Don't worry,
whoo-hoo-hoo-hoo-hoo-hoooooooohhh,
Be happy.
whoo-hoo-hoo-hoo-hoo-hoooooooohhh."

These became some of my favorite songs growing up as a 90's kid living in the 2000's. Mama absolutely loved Prince, so daddy made sure to turn it up a little louder for her. You could hear my mama's faint hums to the song based on how much her nervous system would allow a sound to release. Daddy and I filled in the rest of the notes of each sound with our off-key bellows and jive dance moves.

The most special part about the RV trip was finally getting to lay in bed with my mama. Imagine that for the first time since you were a gabbling, drooling, baby, that you could lie in bed with your mama. You get to personally smell her scent mixed with the scents of hospital pads, plastic of feeding tubes, and a hint of medicated creams. You get to feel her warm almond-cocoa skin on the side of your torso. You hear the pattern of her breath and feel the vibration of her heartbeat—for the first time at age eight. I was overly ecstatic but incredibly nervous for this moment. I wondered how it would feel. Would she be able to feel my body? Would I feel comfortable beside her? Would this feel awkward for me? Would I squish her? Would she squish me? I honestly didn't know what to expect. I hated to have the internal battle of even being nervous about sleeping with my own mama, yet I knew it came with the human territory. The moment was so powerful that it brought small tears in my eyes and palpitations in my heart as I crawled into the bed with her. I cuddled up coldly beside her warm, soft skin. I continued having a bodily response as I laid still and allowed myself to become comfortable. After a short while, I felt the safest I had ever felt in my life. I almost didn't want to leave the bed in the morning. I knew that daddy was worried about how nervous, and almost resistant, I was about sleeping in bed with her. We didn't want mama to think that I was afraid of her. Quite opposing, I was hoping that my presence would be everything that she needed for this RV trip.

As we closed out the final days of the trip, I became a little gloomy in a bittersweet tone. Although I was excited for a new beginning, this once in a lifetime experience was truly over. We wouldn't stop at any more crazy places, sing any more wild songs, or have any more fun and crazy nights. And, I know I couldn't sleep in the bed with mama anymore. It was anxiety-inducing, but I am glad that it happened. It taught me the true power of intimacy. I learned how to be closer to mama in a way that was comfortable for the both of us, but to also be more physically vulnerable with the people I loved. Since mama couldn't hold me or hug me, I learned that I needed to become okay with showing physical affection to her. After all, she is still a human too. Even though this was a very short trip, I knew that this would always be a moment to treasure.

Life is truly a highway.

Mama Loves the Bad Boys

ONE THING THAT MADE THE RELATIONSHIP with mama so unique was that I loved the opportunity to learn more about the things that made mama more human everyday. It was quite easy as a child to slip into a routine of thinking that mama was limited only to certain ideas, feelings, and thoughts. Because she wasn't able to talk or fully express, sometimes it was hard to remember that she still had things that she really liked too. In society, we truly are conditioned to believe that only actions and words make someone fully human, not recognizing the complexity of the human experience. For someone like mama who is missing a layer of expression, it takes a lot more effort to know her and understand who she is and what she likes because she cannot verbally tell you or demonstrate in action. It was honestly an enriching lesson to learn about mama, which carried on into other relationships that I formed. I've learned to see people beyond what they say or do to explore more of who they are. This is what allowed me to connect in a way that is almost indestructible.

Daddy would tell me about the things that she deeply loved when they first met and how it used to drive him crazy that she loved it so much. It was always so beautiful to see a demonstration of true love when daddy would absolutely support the things that mama loved. I loved hearing mama's favorite artists in the car with daddy and how he would play it over and over again. It showed how much he wanted a piece of her with him at all times no matter where he was, and honestly, so did I. Along with mama's passion for certain musical artists, mama also loved particular sports teams as well. Sports have definitely served a special place in her heart so it is always exciting to see mama keep up with something she enjoys. With her passion for good music and for good sports, it always bonded us to watch and listen as a family.

As a family, we are huge Ohio State fans. We wouldn't miss a single Saturday to watch the football games, and daddy made sure that mama caught every women's basketball game possible. When mama was living at the house, daddy would lay an Ohio State towel over her body and put an OSU baseball cap on her head. We would shout, yell, and cheer together through the wins and losses of the season. Sometimes, grandpa would join us in the fun too. It was exciting to know that mama could be so involved in the Ohio State football experience that she planned to do when she was originally in college. This truly became a national holiday in my house every single Saturday during football season. From age three and beyond, I never missed one Ohio State football game, which continued on until I actually attended the school and went to the games in person. These moments definitely ingrained the intense passion to be a Buckeye, which is why I always knew I would graduate from Ohio State many years later. It was special to us all to bond on watching the grittiness of our Buckeyes and go through the emotional stressors over the years. Highlighting some key players like RB Maurice Clarett (02), DB/WR Chris

Gamble (01-03), DB Malcolm Jenkins (05-08), SS Mike Doss (99-02), DE Mike Vrabel (93-96), WR Teddy Ginn Jr (04-06), WR/DB Santonio Holmes (03-06), RB "Beanie" Wells (06-09), LB A. J. Hawk (02-05), and my favorite of all time QB Troy Smith (02-06). We also got to witness one championship as a family, which was back in 2002 in a double OT game against the Miami Hurricanes. It was the most joyful day of our lives, and the second most joyful day as I got to witness a second championship win during my senior year at Ohio State.

A musical icon that mama was absolutely crazy about, and that drove daddy crazy, was the rock/pop legend, Prince. "When Doves Cry", "Diamonds and Pearls", and "Purple Rain" were just a few jams that I heard quite a million times in the house. Daddy said mama also loved Darryl Hall and John Oates, which were these two smooth white men who fooled everyone on the radio because they sounded black. Conclusively, mama was in love with these singers and daddy never understood how. Prince truly had a way with his musicianship, provocative body movements, and explicit lyrics. It was incredible to listen to the types of things he could truly create. With his superb musicianship, Prince also knew how to get all of the ladies, including mama. No matter the moment, if daddy decides to play Prince on TV or on the radio, she will smile from ear to ear with absolutely no shame. It was always rewarding to see more of mama's human response from life. It gave comfort to learn from a woman what attraction looked like and how mama experienced it. There were certain singers and rappers that I thought were cute at the time, so it was fun to see how that manifested within mama. It often was scary thinking on how I would figure out how to address attraction and boys when I didn't exactly have the opportunity to talk about it back and forth with mama. Nonetheless, the type of woman that she was and the way she carried herself showed a strong example on who to become. And, she made it feel human and normal to enjoy diverse people that may not be fully appropriate to some. She liked her boys a little bad, too.

Speaking of "bad boys", as a true basketball player, mama had a favorite NBA team that she would always follow -- the Detroit Pistons, specifically the era of "The Bad Boys". While there were a few transient players on the Pistons team during this time, they primarily consisted of Isaiah Thomas, John

Salley, Dennis Rodman, Ralph Lewis, and Joe Dumars. They were known for being the dirtiest of dirty when it came to aggressively playing ball. This came from an era where the pace of basketball was shifting and there was a lot more diverse talent hitting the courts. Their tactic was to be as gritty and aggressive as possible to throw the opponents off of their game. They were told that if you get a foul, get a good foul. They were able to "fight" themselves into becoming the Eastern Conference Champions. Their games were full of the greatest level of aggression, and mama loved it.

Right along with her (and through pure irony), I was also a fan of the 2000's Detroit Pistons (as well as the Spurs, which is the complete opposite in personality). This team included Chauncey Billups, "Rip" Hamilton, Tayshaun Prince, Rasheed Wallace, and "Big Ben" Wallace. They weren't as bad as the bad boys, but they surely had a lot of aggression that I loved, just like mama. I loved that there was such a strong diversity of skill sets. Billups was an incredible point guard that truly set up each player to become even greater. I learned a lot of my game from the Wallace guys through the use of aggression, intense pace, and skill. It was so exciting to watch how they always came alive. Daddy would make sure that every time the Detroit Pistons played on TV, my mama was watching it. Daddy was not a fan of them at all, because he didn't like all of the unnecessary aggression. Nonetheless, he was a fan of her. When daddy noticed that I also took a liking to the Bad Boys of the Pistons, he couldn't help but roll his eyes. Mama and I would grin together from ear to ear cheering on all of the aggressive, dirty calls and the vulgar gestures from Rasheed Wallace, or the harsh pushes from Big Ben. Even when my mama was in the nursing home, we would make sure that her TV was set to the Pistons game. It was the greatest week ever when we gathered in her half of a room within the nursing home to watch the championship series against the Lakers, ending their dynasty in Game 5. I remember how happy we all were, but daddy and I were especially happy that mama could witness her Bad Boys winning again.

Moments like this often brought alive the idea that without saying a word, without dribbling a ball together, or without any signs, mama was literally within me. To know that we have similar attractions and similar interests in what type of basketball that we enjoy shows how strong a mama's touch will always be without even having to try. When playing ball, it made me more confident to be a little more aggressive because it reflected the players that I admired and it reflected who mama and I loved to watch. I knew that part of me connected me to mama when she played basketball. It was such a unique bond as such that made it an honor to play basketball for her. I often wondered if watching the women playing on TV in the Ohio State games made her think about how she could have played with them if she didn't become ill. I wondered if it made her reflect on her love for the sport. This truly motivated me to honor and uplift how important the sport was to the both of us, and how it brought us both a healthy escape from life. This too also made watching basketball even more special because it was our own way to experience the thing we both love in the best way we knew how. Although the Pistons are not the teams that neither her nor I loved anymore, I do hope to one day carry such a bond down to my offspring.

Growing up with mama disabled meant I had most of my social conversations with daddy. Although daddy was very knowledgeable in a lot of areas of life, talking about boys and attraction will never come off any easier. Daddy had a pretty young girl growing into a woman and his conversation was very daddy-ish to say the least. I often wished that I could have sat with mama and told her about someone who I thought was cute or someone who I liked at school. I even wanted to feel safe saying that I thought Nelly was the finest man I had ever seen as a 6th grader and not feel like I was being "fast" for liking boys. It was also hard to figure out how to navigate flirting, dating, and other romantically involved things when I didn't have mama fully to talk to. Nonetheless, I found comfort in knowing the people who mama was attracted to and found ways to connect with her in that manner. I learned the tenacity to make the most of the things I had and trusting my wisdom for the rest.

I hope to mirror the love mama showed to me that was already placed in my DNA before I was born. I think that this is the most ultimately connecting experience of love that a child can receive, and the most relieving form of love that a mother can give. I hope that I can share similar interests and attractions and make my kids feel safe just because of who I am, and not always based on what I say. My offspring may not like everything or everyone I like, but I do know that we can still have connecting experiences on the things we do love. Truthfully, I cannot wait to share moments like this with my children, without even saying a word. I hope they even feel a part of mama within them.

We love the Bad Boys.

Dear Mama–

Thank you for who you were to me. Although the world may have not fully understood who you were, I thank God for allowing me to have the aligned vision to see every part of your motherhood. Through all of the memories of you, I now see everything that you taught me and every seed that you planted. In fertile soil, I have now rooted in your character, sprouted in your wisdom, and blossomed in your love for others. I can now see who you are within me.

I can only imagine how challenging it was to navigate life with a disability that most struggled to overlook. I could only imagine how it felt to not fully hold your daughter at any given moment, or lay next to your husband when you needed him most. I would predict frustration in wanting to communicate your greatest needs and not being able to physically do so. Yet, I commend you for handling this with grace, peace, and joy. I pray that I continue to embody who you were without the physical and mental advantages of others. I pray that I continue to free your truths from the spaces that once hid them and to walk boldly in everything that you are. I pray I will become the beautiful wife and great mother you were and to experience your guidance along the way. I will continue to be strong, joyful, courageous, loving, creative, unique, and full of voice–because I know that is who you shaped me to become.

I love you, mama.

Love,
April

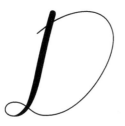R. APRIL BEE IS AN AUTHOR, POET, transformational speaker and wellness coach. Bee is the Founder and Owner of RAW Honey Wellness and Coaching, focusing on the impact of generational trauma on wellness and liberation in black communities. After losing her mother at 14, Bee was inspired to address the impact of trauma on chronic illness, as well as access to adequate wellness education and resources. She hopes to utilize artistic expression, storytelling, and coaching to connect people to the hope in finding healing and purpose for each person who may be impacted by her personal experiences.

Lightning Source UK Ltd.
Milton Keynes UK
UKHW020918260922
409453UK00005B/30